Oral Health Book For Kids

Dental Wellness for Children

Health and Happiness

Dr. Anthony B. Gallagher

Acknowledgment

The method involved with expressing "Oral Health Book For Kids" has been one of motivation, training, and gratitude. I owe an obligation of appreciation to those whose commitments to the area of oral wellbeing have motivated and urged me to undertake this work.

First and foremost, I need to say thanks to Dr. Sarah White for her commitment to paediatric dentistry and her cutting-edge examinations, which have filled me with a consistent wellspring of motivation. Your obligation to assist jokes with keeping up with great oral wellbeing has enlivened me to advance dental health and give them the certainty to deal with their teeth.

I'm extremely enthusiastic about Dr. David Johnson's commitments to safeguarding dentistry. My attention to the worth of early mediation and the role preventive consideration plays in protecting superb oral wellbeing has been formed by your insight and experience.

Also, I need to say thanks to Dr. Emily Brown for her persistent endeavours to instruct families about the significance of practising great dental cleanliness. Your commitment to advancing dental wellbeing has propelled me to foster educational materials that urge children to value their oral wellbeing and adopt great ways of behaving.

I'm extremely appreciative to my family for their steady help and consolation during this excursion, notwithstanding the recognized specialists shown previously. I value your understanding and confidence in my vision, dear spouse Rebecca and my kids Isabella and Ethan. My greatest motivation and wellspring of solidarity have come from your adoration and backing.

I likewise need to thank my folks, John Williamson, for showing me the worth of training and the meaning of being a decent neighbour. I will constantly be energetic about your affection and backing since they assisted me in turning into the individual I am today through your recommendation and understanding.

At last, however, similarly as significantly, I need to offer my thanks to my pursuers in general and allies who have invited "Oral Health Book For Kids ' with great affection and an uplifting perspective. Your remarks and backing want to teach others about oral wellbeing and give kids the instruments they need to take great consideration of their teeth.

I feel truly lucky and humbled to have gotten the opportunity to make "Oral Health Book For Kids ," and I need to offer my thanks to every individual who assisted me in working out. By cooperating, we can make a world in which each youngster can grin with joy and certainty and rouse another generation of dental heroes.

With appreciation

Dr. Antony B. Gallagher

CONTENT

Introduction

Imagine a reality where each kid's grin transmits with certainty, where sparkling teeth and sound gums are the standard as opposed to the special case. Imagine a future where kids embrace dental consideration as a characteristic piece of their day-to-day everyday practice, where visits to the dental specialist are met with fervour as opposed to misgiving. Welcome to the universe of "Oral Health Book For Kids," a progressive manual that engages kids to assume command over their oral wellbeing and set out on an excursion to a long period of sound grins.

In the pages of this book, kids find the sorcery of oral cleanliness through enthralling stories, intelligent riddles, and exciting games. From the second they open the cover, they are shipped into an existence where toothbrushes become superheroes, dental floss changes into a mysterious string, and solid propensities lead to stunning grins.

In any case, "Oral Health Book For Kids" is something other than an assortment of dental tips and tricks—it's an exhaustive manual for grasping the significance of oral wellbeing and developing deep-rooted propensities that advance dental health. Through drawing in accounts and engaging characters, kids find out about the life structures of the mouth, the role of diet in dental wellbeing, and the meaning of ordinary dental check-ups.

The excursion starts with "Brushing Nuts and Bolts," where kids are acquainted with the basics of legitimate brushing methods and the significance of everyday oral consideration. As they turn the pages, they set out on an undertaking to investigate the "Portions of the Mouth," finding the one-of-a-kind elements of every tooth and the job they play in keeping a solid grin.

Yet, the fervour doesn't stop there—kids jump further into the universe of oral wellbeing as they uncover "Fun Realities About Teeth and Oral Cleanliness." From the secrets of tooth finish to the amazing advantages of spit, they uncover a gold mine of intriguing data that starts their interest and lights their energy for dental wellbeing.

As they explore through the pages of "Oral Health Book For Kids," kids experience difficulties and obstructions that test their insight and critical thinking abilities. They tackle tests, address perplexities, and participate in intuitive games that build up key ideas and develop how they might interpret oral cleanliness.

In any case, maybe the most remarkable part of this book is its capacity to move and persuade kids to take responsibility for their oral wellbeing. Through moving stories and inspiring messages, youngsters discover that they have the ability to safeguard their grins and shield their prosperity. They find that dental consideration isn't just about brushing and flossing; it's tied in with supporting an uplifting outlook towards taking care of oneself and embracing the magnificence of a solid grin.

At its centre, "Oral Health Book For Kids" is a source of inspiration—a mobilising sob for kids wherever to focus on their oral wellbeing and set out on an excursion to a more splendid, better future. It's a demonstration of the groundbreaking force of information and the significant effect that little activities can have on our lives.

So go along with us on this experience—jam into the pages of "Oral Health Book For Kids" and open the key to a long period of sound grins. Together, we can rouse another age of dental heroes and make an existence where each youngster can grin with certainty and euphoria.

What is oral health?

The condition of the mouth, which incorporates the teeth, gums, tongue, and other oral designs, as well as the overall soundness of these parts, is referred to as oral wellbeing. It incorporates various variables, including capability, cleanliness, and the absence of diseases or issues in the oral cavity.

In spite of the fact that they are huge variables, having a brilliant grin and new breath are not by any means the only parts of oral wellbeing. It additionally incorporates keeping up with the mouth's typical capability, which is fundamental for essential capabilities like eating, talking, and, in any event, communicating feelings with looks.

Supporting ideal dental well-being is critical for general prosperity and life fulfilment. Since the mouth fills in as the body's entry, oral medical conditions might have a foundational influence and fuel other medical conditions that don't just influence the mouth. Gum illness, for example, has been associated with respiratory contamination, diabetes, and coronary illness.

Various factors, like individual propensities, way of life choices, hereditary inclinations, and availability of dental treatment, influence oral wellbeing. Keeping up with ideal oral wellbeing requires rehearsing suitable oral cleanliness rehearsals, like brushing and flossing consistently, eating a reasonable eating routine low in sweet and acidic food sources, and going to the dental specialist for exams and cleanings.

Babies and teens ought to likewise be worried about their dental wellbeing, notwithstanding adults. A long period of sound teeth and gums is based on the early reception of proper oral cleanliness rehearsals. By showing kids great oral cleanliness propensities and ensuring they seek dental treatment on time, guardians and different parental figures might assist jokes around with keeping up with great oral wellbeing.

Oral wellbeing is an expansive term that incorporates the condition of the mouth and its constituent parts, as well as their working, tidiness, and general prosperity. Keeping up with it requires a blend of individual endeavours, great ways of behaving, and admission to dental consideration. General wellbeing and personal satisfaction are fundamental.

Why is oral health important?

Keeping your mouth solid is significant for some reasons, more than just having a perfect, white grin and new breath. Our oral wellbeing altogether affects our overall wellbeing and delight throughout everyday life.

As a matter of some importance, our ability to eat and value food is significantly impacted by our dental wellbeing. The most common way of separating food into more modest pieces for simple gulping and absorption begins in the mouth with our teeth. We can appropriately bite food on the off chance that we have solid teeth and gums, which is essential for both ideal nourishment and happiness regarding a changed and even eating regimen.

Past the functional side of eating, there are major areas of strength for dental and actual wellbeing. A huge number of microscopic organisms live in the mouth; some are useful, yet others might be perilous whenever given the opportunity to become uncontrolled. Dismissing oral cleanliness might make microorganisms develop on the gums and teeth, which can bring about the advancement of plaque and tartar. Gum illness, tooth rot, and other oral infections might result from this after some time.

Various fundamental medical problems, including diabetes, respiratory contamination, cardiovascular illness, and troublesome pregnancy results, have been associated with unfortunate oral wellbeing. Analysts have found connections between irritation in the mouth and different locales of the body, showing that fundamental wellbeing and complete degrees of aggravation might be affected by dental wellbeing.

Oral wellbeing has social and mental consequences, notwithstanding the actual ones. A wonderful, solid grin might increase self-esteem and certainty, making it simpler for individuals to draw in with others in a loose and sure way. Then again, dental issues like pits, unfortunate breath, or missing teeth might be humiliating and trashed by society, which causes individuals to feel hesitant and alone.

Moreover, creating solid dental propensities as a youth might take care of you sometime down the road, even into adulthood.

Adolescents who seek standard dental treatment and are shown great oral cleanliness propensities are bound to stay with them all through their lives, which brings down their opportunity to later have dental issues.

By and large, it is difficult to underscore how significant dental wellbeing is. It assumes a significant role in our overall well being and prosperity, influencing our actual wellbeing as well as our personal satisfaction, social connections, and fearlessness. We can safeguard our oral wellbeing and get its various benefits by focusing on oral tidiness and booking routine dental treatment.

Fun facts about teeth and oral hygiene

We ought to examine a couple of spellbinding and fascinating real factors that could stun and engage you about teeth and oral prosperity!

We all have particular teeth and fingerprints; did you have any idea about that? No two people have a similar arrangement of teeth, similar to fingerprints. In view of their uniqueness, dental records are a valuable asset for individual recognition in measurable examinations.

With regards to singularity, did you have any idea that the human teeth are the main substantial parts unequipped for self-mending? Teeth can't recharge or retouch all alone, in contrast to bones or skin. It is crucial to take legitimate care of them by brushing, flossing, and seeing the dental specialist consistently.

Teeth have astounding strength! Perhaps the hardest material in the human body—much harder than bone—iis polish, which covers most of the teeth. Teeth are solid; however, they are not rugged; outrageous power or rot might in any case hurt.

Have you at any point asked why people just at any point have two arrangements of teeth? Close to a half-year-old enough, the principal set of teeth, at times called child or essential teeth, start to eject. Around age six, super-durable teeth start to supplant the principal set of teeth dynamically. Most adults have 32 long-lasting teeth when they are adults, four of which are astute teeth.

In related news, did you have any idea that not every person gets shrewd teeth? While certain people might have one, two, three, or every one of the four insight teeth upon entering the world, others may not. Insightful tooth extraction might be important because of issues including impaction, swarming, or disease.

Fun reality: there are more than 300 distinct sorts of microscopic organisms tracked down in dental plaque, the tacky film that develops on teeth! On the off chance that incessant brushing and flossing are not finished to dispose of these microscopic organisms, which are benefited from sugars and starches from our feasts, they can create acids that might disintegrate tooth veneer and cause depressions.

Do you have any idea what "dental floss movements" are? By adding engaging music and moving developments to their oral hygiene strategies, a few dental specialists have concocted inventive techniques to inspire children to floss. These engaging activities not only assist with making lifetime propensities for legitimate dental cleanliness, yet they likewise make flossing more lovely.

Not in the least do non-human creatures wash their teeth; were you aware? Certain creatures, such as a few sorts of chimpanzees, elephants, and monkeys, have been seen cleaning their teeth with sticks or twigs. What about working on dental cleanliness to an unheard-of level?

The interesting and different field of dental wellbeing is highlighted by these engaging realities about teeth and oral cleanliness. There's continuously something new and captivating to find out about our teeth, whether it's respecting the constancy of lacquer, grasping the nuances of dental plaque, or seeing uncommon propensities in the creature domain.

Parts of the Mouth

We should investigate the numerous and fascinating parts of the mouth, every one of which is vital for our ability to eat, talk, and communicate our thoughts.

Above all else, with regards to eating and separating food, teeth are the superstars. Grown-ups ordinarily have 32 teeth, which incorporate incisors, canines, premolars, and molars. Each sort of tooth has an unmistakable reason for biting, going from gnawing and tearing to smashing and crushing.

Then, we have the gingiva, or gums, which are the supporting tissues that surround and secure our teeth. Keeping up with solid gums is critical for safeguarding the dependability and arrangement of teeth as well as protecting the fundamental bone construction from damage or contamination.

Then, we should discuss the tongue, a muscle that serves as a strong, tangible organ that guides discourse and taste discernment. The tongue is covered with little taste buds that empower us to recognize various preferences, including sweet, harsh, pungent, and severe. The tongue is fundamental for creating talking sounds and helping with gulping, notwithstanding taste.

The sense of taste, which is the top of the mouth isolated into the hard sense of taste at the front and the delicate sense of taste at the back, ought not be disregarded. While the delicate sense of taste supports fixing up the nasal entries during gulping to hold food or liquids back from entering the nose, the hard sense of taste offers serious areas of strength for the tongue to press against while biting.

The uvula, a little, plump tissue that stretches out from the delicate sense of taste, is the next organ to arrive at the throat. The uvula is believed to be engaged with gulping, discourse enunciation, and the creation of specific sounds in different dialects, but its exact contribution to these cycles isn't altogether known.

Not to be disregarded are the salivary organs, which give spit, the body's regular mouth grease. Spit incorporates catalysts that separate carbs and lipids to begin the course of absorption and, furthermore, assists with saturating food, making it simpler to swallow. Spit additionally contributes to general oral wellbeing by cleaning the mouth of microbes and food particles.

These many mouth sorts work out to make a complex and intertwined framework that empowers people to complete important undertakings like talking, eating, and self-articulation. The astounding construction and capacities of the human mouth are highlighted by the particular and significant jobs that every part performs.

How each part contributes to oral health

The unmistakable obligations and capabilities that every part of the mouth plays in protecting a splendid and sound grin, as well as how every region of the mouth adds to our general oral wellbeing.

In the first place, teeth are imperative for biting and separating food, however they likewise have a significant capability in safeguarding the respectability of the jawbone. The hidden bone may steadily start to fall apart whenever teeth are lost or taken out, changing the state of the face and maybe presenting wellbeing dangers to oral wellbeing. Thus, keeping teeth looking great is vital for keeping up with the arrangement and capability of the mouth as well as the encompassing bone construction.

How about we continue on toward the gums. They work as a safeguard encompassing the teeth, keeping food particles and microorganisms out of the dissemination and forestalling irritation or contamination. Healthy, the gums are pink, firm, and structure a tight seal around the teeth to assist with forestalling microorganisms. In any case, when gums become excited or contaminated due to terrible dental cleanliness rehearses or different reasons, it might bring about gum sickness, which is a pervasive oral ailment that, whenever left untreated, can prompt gum downturn, tooth misfortune, and, surprisingly, foundational medical problems.

Moreover, the tongue is fundamental for keeping up with dental wellbeing since it goes about as a characteristic mouth cleaner, eliminating microbes and food particles that might cause plaque and foul breath. The tongue likewise works with the suitable conveyance of spit all through the mouth, which helps with absorption and jam the perfect proportion of dampness. Keeping up with great tongue cleanliness, which incorporates routine brushing and scratching, may assist with halting the development of microorganisms and lower the possibility of creating oral medical issues.

Presently we should discuss the sense of taste and that it is so critical to dental wellbeing since it makes talking and gulping simpler. While the delicate sense of taste supports fixing up the nasal entries during gulping to hold food or liquids back from entering the nose, the hard sense of taste offers a firm surface for the tongue to lean against while biting and talking. Keeping up with the most ideal dental well being and staying away from issues like gulping issues or discourse disabilities need appropriate sense of taste capability.

The emission of spit, which fills in as the body's normal safeguard against oral microorganisms and plaque aggregation, is worked with by the salivary organs. Spit helps wash away food particles and microorganisms that might cause depressions and gum infection, kill oral acids, and remineralize tooth veneer. Supporting a solid oral climate and deflecting oral medical conditions like tooth rot and dry mouth need sufficient spit creation.

Each part of the mouth has a unique and fundamental capability to play in advancing our overall oral wellbeing and prosperity. Each component — from the tongue and sense of taste to the salivary organs, teeth, and gums — coopers agreeably to safeguard a brilliant and solid grin. We might ensure the solidness and liveliness of our oral wellbeing into the indefinite future by monitoring the jobs played by every part and by keeping up with suitable oral cleanliness rehearses.

Brushing Basics

Cleaning our teeth is perhaps one of the main propensities we can develop for maintaining ideal oral wellbeing. Besides the fact that it helps eliminate food particles and plaque from the surfaces of our teeth, it likewise forestalls depression, gum sickness, and awful breath.

When it comes to brushing essentials, technique is critical. Utilising a delicately seethed toothbrush and fluoride toothpaste, we ought to clean our teeth tenderly yet completely, covering all surfaces, including the front, back, and biting surfaces of the teeth. It's essential to brush for no less than two minutes, two times per day, preferably once in the first part of the day and once before bed.

The legitimate brushing method includes holding the toothbrush at a 45-degree point to the gums and utilising delicate, roundabout movements to independently brush every tooth. Giving close consideration to regions where plaque will in general amass, for example, along the gumline in the middle between teeth, is fundamental for successful plaque expulsion and preventing gum sickness.

Cleaning the teeth means a lot to brush the tongue and top of the mouth to eliminate microorganisms and renew breath. A few toothbrushes even include an inherent tongue scrubber on the rear of the brush head for this reason.

Selecting the right toothbrush and toothpaste is critical for successful brushing. While manual and rotating brushes are both successful at eliminating plaque, certain individuals might find rotating brushes more straightforward to utilise, particularly those with ability issues or supports. With respect to toothpaste, fluoride toothpaste is prescribed for its capacity to reinforce tooth veneers and forestall cavities.

Actually, important brushing alone isn't sufficient to keep up with ideal oral wellbeing. Flossing every day and utilising mouthwash can assist with eliminating plaque and microorganisms from regions that brushing might miss, such as the middle of the teeth and along the gumline. Furthermore, ordinary dental check-ups and cleanings are fundamental for identifying and preventing oral medical problems before they worsen.

Brushing fundamentals are fundamental for keeping up with ideal oral wellbeing and preventing normal dental issues like pits, gum infections, and terrible breath. By embracing the appropriate brushing method, picking the right devices, and integrating flossing and mouthwash into our oral hygiene schedule, we can guarantee the wellbeing and life span of our grins long into the future.

The importance of brushing

Cleaning our teeth is something beyond a regular undertaking; it's the establishment for keeping up with real oral cleanliness and staying away from dental issues. It is difficult to misshape how important brushing is for keeping food particles, microorganisms, and plaque off our teeth's surfaces, which helps us stay away from despondencies, gum disease, and other oral clinical issues.

Plaque, a shabby layer of microorganisms that accumulates on teeth throughout the day, is the essential driver of various dental issues. Plaque could become tartar, a hard, yellowish covering that should be taken out by a dental expert in case it isn't cleared out by progressive brushing and flossing. At the point when left untreated, tartar assortment along the gum line might prompt gum disease, a ceaseless oral clinical issue portrayed by kicking the bucket, red, expanded gums, and perhaps a tooth incident.

As well as hindering gum disease and holes, brushing invigorates breath by cleaning the mouth of microorganisms that cause aroma. Halitosis, or horrendous breath, may be upsetting and socially wrong, which can antagonistically influence our certainty and social affiliations. Normal brushing, tongue scratching, and mouthwash utilization help to maintain a magnificent, new breath every day of the week.

Moreover, brushing is fundamental for saving the decency of our tooth facade, which is the hard outside covering of our teeth. Acidic food sources and drinks, as well as the acids made by oral microorganisms, may crumble. Fluoride toothpaste decreases the pace of despondency and dental responsiveness by keeping teeth clean and defending them from destructive breaking down.

Brushing influences our general flourishing, despite its nearby impact on dental prosperity. Studies have shown links between central clinical issues, including diabetes, coronary ailment, respiratory defilement, and sad dental prosperity. By rehearsing authentic dental cleanliness, for instance, brushing reliably, we could lessen the chance of getting these and other clinical issues.

Besides, brushing is a fundamental piece of our everyday dealing with ourselves schedule, as it develops sensations of sureness, orderliness, and freshness. Having an unbelievable, strong grin could assist us with having a superior point of view toward ourselves and our point of interaction with others even more. Also, it gives us the assurance to chuckle, smile, and talk.

Distorting the advantages of brushing is unfathomable. It is a key piece of fitting oral cleanliness and is basic for avoiding dental issues, further creating breath, and developing general prosperity and thriving. We can guarantee the prosperity and strength of our teeth for quite a while by making progressive dental check-ups, brushing, flossing, and mouthwash usage a necessity.

How to brush properly

Proper brushing technique is critical in order to maintain good oral health, avoid dental issues, and remove plaque, germs, and food particles from our teeth's surfaces. Let's examine the essential elements of a correct brushing technique to guarantee a deep and efficient cleaning.

The most crucial thing to remember is to use the appropriate equipment for the task. A toothbrush with soft bristles, a compact head, and a comfortable grip is the best choice for cleaning every part of the mouth, including the hard-to-reach places between teeth and along the gum line. Furthermore, since fluoride toothpaste strengthens tooth enamel and prevents cavities, it is advised to use it.

When it comes to brushing technique, the first step is to place the toothbrush so that it is at a 45-degree angle to the gums. This enables the bristles to penetrate below the gum line, where germs and plaque often build up. Brush each tooth separately, making sure to cover the chewing, front, and back surfaces with soft, circular movements. Pay special attention to regions like the spaces between teeth and the gum line, where plaque is more likely to build up.

Brushing should be done for two minutes at least twice a day, preferably in the morning and just before bed. To make sure you're brushing for the correct amount of time, set a timer or turn on the music. Refrain from cleaning your teeth too hard, as this might erode the enamel and cause gum irritation.

Rather, to properly remove plaque without harming the teeth or gums, employ soft, controlled movements.

To get rid of germs and freshen your breath, remember to brush your tongue and the roof of your mouth in addition to your teeth. To gently remove dirt and germs from the tongue's surface, some toothbrushes include a built-in tongue scraper on the rear of the brush head.

You might think about adding mouthwash and flossing to your regular oral hygiene routine to get the most out of your brushing sessions. Flossing helps get rid of food particles and plaque from places that brushing could miss, such as the spaces between teeth and the gum line. Mouthwash offers an extra line of defence against issues with oral health by helping to wash away any leftover germs and refresh breath.

Remember to change your toothbrush every three to four months, or more often if the bristles start to fray or show signs of wear. A dirty toothbrush harbours germs and is less efficient at eliminating plaque, which raises the possibility of oral health issues.

Using the right brushing method is crucial to preserving good oral health and averting dental issues. A comprehensive and efficient cleaning that supports a bright, healthy smile for years to come may be achieved by selecting the appropriate brushes, brushing for the prescribed amount of time, and using gentle, circular strokes.

Choosing the right toothbrush and toothpaste

Choosing the right toothbrush and toothpaste is vital for maintaining ideal oral wellbeing and guaranteeing a successful brushing schedule. With a wide array of choices accessible, picking the best items for your singular needs can be overwhelming. We should investigate the variables to consider while choosing the right toothbrush and toothpaste for you.

With regards to picking a toothbrush, there are a few variables to consider, including the size, shape, and fibre type. Deciding on a toothbrush with a little, conservative head considers more straightforward mobility and access to hard-to-arrive-at regions of the mouth, like the back molars. Furthermore, choosing a toothbrush with delicate fibres is suggested, as they are delicate on the gums and tooth finish, decreasing the risk of irritation or harm.

Another consideration is whether to use a manual or oscillating brush. The two kinds of toothbrushes can actually eliminate plaque and microbes when utilised appropriately, so the choice eventually boils down to individual inclination. Certain individuals might find rotating brushes simpler to utilise, particularly for those with mastery issues or supports, as they give a more steady brushing movement and may offer extra highlights like clocks or tension sensors.

Choosing the right toothpaste is similarly significant for maintaining ideal oral wellbeing. While picking a toothpaste, search for one that contains fluoride, a mineral that reinforces tooth polish and prevents holes. Fluoride toothpaste is essential for protecting against corrosive disintegration and keeping teeth honest.

Past fluoride, there are different sorts of toothpaste accessible to address explicit oral wellbeing needs. For instance, toothpaste figured out for delicate teeth contains fixings that assist with desensitising the teeth and diminish inconvenience brought about by hot or cold temperatures. Brightening toothpaste contains rough particles or compound specialists that assist with eliminating surface stains and lightening the teeth over the long haul.

For those with explicit dental worries, for example, gum illness or dry mouth, there are toothpastes accessible that are exceptionally figured out to resolve these issues. These toothpastes may contain extra fixings, such as antibacterial specialists or lotions, to help improve gum health or reduce dry mouth side effects.

The best toothbrush and toothpaste for you depends on your unique necessities, inclinations, and oral wellbeing objectives. It's critical to pick items that you feel happy utilising and that successfully address your particular worries. By choosing the right toothbrush and toothpaste and integrating them into your everyday oral hygiene schedule, you can keep up with ideal oral wellbeing and partake in a sound, energetic grin for quite a long time into the future.

Flossing Fun

Flossing may not generally be the most thrilling piece of our everyday daily practice, yet it assumes a critical role in eliminating plaque, food particles, and microbes from regions that brushing alone may miss, in the middle among teeth and along the gumline. By flossing routinely, we can forestall pits, gum infections, and terrible breath, guaranteeing a sound, energetic grin.

Anyway, how might we make flossing more tomfoolery and locking in? One way is to integrate music or a favourite webcast into your flossing schedule. Standing by and listening to cherry tunes or a fascinating digital broadcast episode can assist with relaxing and occupying any uneasiness or dreariness related to flossing.

Another thought is to transform flossing into a social movement by flossing with an accomplice or relative. In addition to the fact that this gives you responsibility and inspiration to adhere to your flossing schedule, it also permits you to bond and associate with friends and family while dealing with your oral wellbeing together.

For the individuals who partake in a touch of contest, consider transforming flossing into a game or challenge. Put forth objectives or achievements for yourself, for example, flossing consistently for a month or evaluating various sorts of floss to see which one you like best. You could make a prize framework for arriving at your flossing objectives, for example, by indulging yourself in an exceptional treat or action.

Get inventive with your flossing routine by evaluating different flossing apparatuses and procedures. Customary dental floss is only one choice; there are also floss picks, interdental brushes, and water flossers accessible that might be more agreeable or advantageous for you. Try different things with various flossing apparatuses to find the one that turns out best for your singular necessities and inclinations.

Transform flossing into a care practice by zeroing in on the sensations and developments of flossing as you make it happen. Focus on how the floss coasts between your teeth and the sensation of neatness and newness a while later.

Integrating care into your flossing routine can assist you with developing a more prominent feeling of mindfulness and appreciation for this significant oral cleanliness propensity.

Remember to commend your flossing victories and achievements en route. Whether it's finishing a flossing challenge, evaluating a new flossing strategy, or absolutely adhering to your flossing routine reliably, invest heavily in your endeavours and accomplishments. Recall that each time you floss, you're making a significant stride towards keeping up with ideal oral wellbeing and guaranteeing a sound, cheerful grin into the indefinite future.

Flossing may not generally be the most thrilling piece of our day-to-day everyday practice, except that it's a fundamental propensity for keeping up with ideal oral wellbeing. By consolidating music, associating gamification, inventiveness, care, and festivity into our flossing schedule, we can make this significant undertaking more charming and successful, guaranteeing a sound, energetic grin forever.

Why flossing is essential

Flossing is a fundamental piece of a careful oral hygiene routine; it isn't just a discretionary extension of brushing. Brushing is a superb method for eliminating microorganisms and plaque from the surfaces of your teeth, yet it can't get into the little holes between your teeth and along your gum line, which is where plaque will develop in general. Flossing is helpful in this present circumstance.

By reliably flossing, we may effectively dispense with microorganisms, food particles, and plaque from these challenging-to-arrive-at places, stopping the advancement of gum illness, holes, and foul breath. On the off chance that flossing isn't done accurately, plaque might amass in the spaces between teeth and along the gum line. On the off chance that this isn't tended to, it can cause disease, irritation, and, at last, tooth misfortune.

Periodontal infection, one more name for gum illness, is a far-reaching oral medical problem that influences a large number of people internationally. Whenever left untreated, gum disease, which is described by red, enlarged, and promptly draining gums, may form into additional serious kinds of periodontitis. By killing microorganisms and plaque from the gum line and staying away from the development of tartar—a solidified kind of plaque that must be eliminated by a dental specialist—FFlossing is vital for preventing gum illness.

Furthermore, various fundamental medical problems, including diabetes, lung contamination, and coronary illness, have been associated with gum sickness. The microorganisms that cause gum infection can go all through the body and enter the circulatory system, causing aggravation and raising the risk of these and other diseases. Normal flossing might help protect our overall wellbeing and prosperity by staying away from gum sickness.

Moreover, protecting new breath and keeping away from halitosis, or foul breath, rely upon flossing. The creation of putrid gases by food particles and microbes caught among teeth and along the gum line might prompt awful breath. We might dispose of these scent-causing compounds and keep up with new, wonderful breath the entire day by flossing consistently.

Flossing is fundamental for keeping up with the underlying respectability of the teeth and surrounding tissues. Unrestrained plaque and bacterial gathering may ultimately cause tooth rot, gum downturn, and, surprisingly, bone misfortune. Flossing guarantees the wellbeing and life expectancy of our grins by taking out the synthetics that lead to the advancement of these issues.

Keeping up with great oral wellbeing and staying away from dental issues like holes, gum sickness, and unfortunate breath need customary flossing. Flossing keeps up with our teeth, gums, and general wellbeing for a long period of good grins by eliminating plaque, food particles, and microbes from hard-to-arrive at districts among teeth and along the gumline.

Step-by-step guide to flossing

Let's examine the flossing procedure step-by-step, dissecting each action to guarantee a comprehensive and efficient cleaning regimen.

Step 1: Begin by ripping out an 18- to 24-inch length of dental floss. This guarantees that you have adequate length to work with and enables you to use a new portion of floss for every tooth.

Step 2: With one to two inches of floss remaining between your thumbs and index fingers, hold the floss in place. To guide the floss and adjust the tension, use your thumbs and index fingers.

Step 3: Use a back-and-forth motion to guide the floss under the gum line as you gently glide it between two teeth. It might irritate or hurt, so take care not to snap the floss against the gums.

Step 4: After the floss is below the gum line, gently move it up and down the side of the tooth in a C-shaped curve around one of the teeth. To clean both surfaces of the neighbouring tooth of plaque and debris, repeat this motion.

Step 5: Using the same back-and-forth motion, carefully remove the floss from between the teeth, being cautious not to injure the gums. To prevent germs from moving from one tooth to another, use a new piece of floss for every tooth.

Step 6: Keep flossing every tooth in the mouth, being sure to get behind the final teeth and the rear molars. Pay special attention to regions like the spaces between teeth and the gum line where plaque tends to collect.

Step 7: To get rid of any last bits of floss or germs, give your mouth a good rinse with water. To offer one more line of defense against plaque and foul breath, use mouthwash.

Step 8: Put the used floss in the garbage for disposal. Refrain from disposing of it in the toilet since it may lead to environmental contamination or plumbing issues.

Step 9: To maintain good oral health and avoid dental issues, repeat the flossing procedure at least once a day, preferably just before bed. Plaque and other particles may be loosened by flossing before brushing, which improves toothpaste penetration.

Step 10: In order to maintain the health and lifespan of your smile, remember to combine your flossing regimen with periodic dental examinations and cleanings. Personalised guidance and suggestions from your dentist may be given based on your particular oral health requirements.

Flossing is a little but crucial part of keeping your mouth healthy. This comprehensive flossing instruction can help you maintain a healthy, bright smile for years to come.

Simply follow the steps and include flossing in your regular dental hygiene practice.

Tips to make flossing easier and more enjoyable

We should take a gander at some valuable guidance that will make flossing more pleasurable and easier, so you can without much of a stretch incorporate this significant dental hygiene practice into your day-to-day daily schedule.

1. **Select the suitable flossing executes:** evaluate numerous sorts of flossing carries out to see which one suits you the best. For individuals who experience difficulty utilising customary dental floss, floss picks and interdental brushes are simple substitutes that come in different thicknesses and surfaces. For individuals who wear orthodontic hardware or have

touchy gums, water flossers may likewise be a useful instrument.

2. Set the temperament: light a fragrant candle, turn down the lights, or play quiet music to create a quiet climate that is ideally suited for flossing. You could find it less difficult to incorporate flossing into your everyday practice on the off chance that you make it a wonderful and relaxing experience.

3. Floss while taking part in another action: By joining two errands into one, flossing may turn out to be to a lesser degree a task and a greater amount of productive utilisation of your time. Have a go at flossing while you get up to speed with your most loved book recording, sit in front of the television, or pay attention to a webcast. This allows you to complete your dental consideration routine and focus on something fun.

4. Floss with a companion or relative: Sharing the experience and responsibility of keeping up with your flossing timetable could emerge from flossing with a companion or relative. What's more, it's a brilliant chance to keep up with your dental wellbeing and reinforce your associations with loved ones.

5. Make it a game: By laying out targets or difficulties for oneself, you might make flossing a pleasant and enrapturing exercise. For a month, have a go at flossing every day or try different things with other flossing strategies or supplies. You may likewise plan an arrangement of remunerations for yourself when you achieve your flossing goals, such as giving yourself an extraordinary movement or treat.

6. Utilise enhanced floss: Dental floss is accessible in a range of tastes, including organic products, mint, and cinnamon. It very well may be more pleasant to floss and leave your mouth feeling perfect and new on the off chance that you pick a taste that you like.

7. Be delicate: To forestall disturbance or agony, consistently floss softly as opposed to snapping the floss on your gums. To delicately and effortlessly eliminate plaque, flotsam, and jetsam from teeth and the gum line, utilise slow, intentional developments with the floss.

8. Take part in care work: Focus on the activities and sensations of flossing as you come, and focus on how perfect and invigorated you feel a short time later. Adding care to your flossing practice will assist you in fostering a more profound appreciation for this vital dental wellbeing practice.

9. Honour your achievements: Show that you've had a great time with the work you've done and recognize your achievements as you go. Compliment yourself on keeping up with your dental wellbeing and perceive your achievements, whether it's completing a flossing challenge, endeavouring a new flossing strategy, or simply keeping up with your normal flossing plan.

You might guarantee a sound, brilliant grin for quite a long time into the future by adding these plans to your flossing routine and making it more tomfoolery. Review that keeping a reliable flossing routine is fundamental for achieving better dental wellbeing and general prosperity.

Healthy Habits

Advancing deep-rooted dental wellbeing and prosperity in kids requires laying out great oral hygiene rehearses from an early age. We give youngsters the instruments they need to assume responsibility for their oral wellbeing and structure deep-rooted propensities by showing them the benefit of taking great consideration of their teeth and gums.

Customary tooth brushing is one of the main sound propensities for kids to create. Urge children to utilise a delicately shuddered toothbrush and fluoride toothpaste two times every day, in a perfect world, in the first part of the day and not long before bed. Show them the right brushing strategy, which includes utilising delicate, round strokes to clean the front, back, and biting surfaces of the teeth. Permitting youngsters to pick the flavour of their toothpaste and toothbrush or playing their number one music while they brush might make brushing pleasant.

Train kids on the benefits of flossing consistently to dispose of food particles and plaque from the spaces between their teeth and the gum line. Children might find flossing troublesome, so be patient and give assistance or management as expected until they get the smoothness and coordination important to autonomously perform it. To make flossing less difficult and more diversion for youngsters, have a go at using kid-accommodating flossers or floss picks.

Urge youngsters to consume a decent eating routine loaded with natural products, vegetables, complete grains, and lean meats to assist with maintaining oral wellbeing. Confine the utilisation of sweet bites and beverages, since they might demolish dental pits and rot. Train youngsters to pick milk or water over sugar-filled soft drinks or natural juices. Show kids the benefit of drinking water the entire day to assist with keeping their teeth and gums hydrated and to assist with washing away food particles and microbes from their mouths.

An ordinary dental specialist arrangement is likewise urgent to safeguarding youngsters' oral wellbeing. When a youngster's most memorable tooth arises or around their most memorable birthday, make semiannual dental visits for them. Normal assessments empower the dental specialist to follow the turn of events and development of the youngster's teeth, spot any issues from the beginning, and give deterrent consideration and medicines as required. During their dental arrangements, urge children to voice any different kinds of feedback they might have to fabricate entrust and an open line of correspondence with their oral medical services subject matter experts.

Set a positive example for others by rehearsing legitimate dental cleanliness in your everyday exercises. Since youngsters get the most from individuals in their current circumstances, it is essential to make brushing and flossing a family activity and to exhibit to them the value of good dental cleanliness. To support positive routines and advance consistency, give young people stickers, acclaim, or little snacks for their endeavours in dealing with their teeth and gums.

Be thoughtful and empowering as children foster great dental cleanliness rehearses. For young people to become capable of brushing and flossing and to incorporate these propensities into their day-to-day schedules, it calls for investment and practice. As required, offer help, headings, and delicate updates; additionally, recognize and commend their achievements as they go. By cultivating great dental practices in youngsters at an early age, we set them up

for a long period of wonderful grins and
general wellbeing.

The role of diet in oral health

Diet intricately affects oral wellbeing, influencing the state of our teeth, gums, and oral cavity in general. As well as affecting the development and trustworthiness of our dental designs, what we eat and drink is likewise vital in staying away from dental diseases and saving great oral wellbeing, however long our lives might last.

Most importantly, keeping up with the development and improvement of solid teeth and gums requires an eating regimen that is both adjusted and supplement-rich. Food varieties high in fundamental minerals, including calcium, phosphorus, and vitamin D, are particularly significant for keeping up with bone thickness in the jaw and reinforcing tooth finish. Dairy items, salad greens, and invigorated dinners are great sources of calcium, which fortifies the dental finish and safeguards against holes and rot. Meat, fish, eggs, and dairy items contain phosphorus, which joins with calcium to remineralize tooth enamel and stop disintegration. The body utilises vitamin D, which might be procured by means of diet—like greasy fish, eggs, and braced food varieties—and sun exposure to assist with retaining calcium and keeping up with sound bones.

Our dental wellbeing might be directly influenced by various dinners and beverages. Candy, pop, natural product juices, sports drinks, and other sweet and acidic food varieties and refreshments might take care of oral microorganisms to create acids that disintegrate tooth lacquer, prompting tooth rot and disintegration. Over the long run, eating sweet or acidic food sources and drinks constantly could raise your possibility of developing depression, gum sickness, and other dental issues. Accordingly, it's significant to polish off specific feasts and beverages with some restraint and, where achievable, pick better substitutes.

Food sources high in fibre, such as organic products, vegetables, and whole grains, are additionally really great for your teeth. These dinners increase salivation, which helps wash away microbes and food particles from the mouth, reestablish dental finish, and balance out acidic mouthwash.

Crunchy products of the soil, including celery, carrots, and apples, can work as regular toothbrushes by cleaning tooth surfaces and empowering salivation.

One more significant part of sustenance and dental wellbeing is hydration. Water utilisation over the course of the day hydrates oral cavity tissues, keeps spit creation at its ideal, and washes away microorganisms and food particles from the mouth. Since spit greases up the mouth, supports acids, and prepares for gum illness and tooth rot, it is fundamental for keeping up with oral wellbeing. Thus, it means a lot to drink enough water to keep your mouth sound and keep away from a dry mouth, which raises your possibility of developing dental issues.

Oral wellbeing may likewise be influenced by dinner and bite time and recurrence. Over the course of the day, eating frequently or drinking sweet or acidic beverages opens the teeth to broadened corrosive attacks, which raises the risk of pits and finish debasement. Rather, really try to eat even dinners and snacks consistently, and shun brushing or eating in the middle of feasts. Assuming you should nibble, pick quality food varieties like cheddar, yoghourt, almonds, or crude veggies. You ought to likewise hydrate to assist with washing away food particles and keep your mouth sound.

It is unquestionable that sustenance has an impact on oral wellbeing since food choices directly affect the state of our teeth, gums, and oral cavity overall. We might keep up with ideal oral wellbeing and stay away from dental issues for a long period of sound grins by eating a reasonable, supplement-heavy eating routine that is low in sugar and sharpness, drinking enough water, and embracing careful dietary patterns.

Foods that are good and bad for teeth

Find which food varieties might help or damage your dental wellbeing, what they mean for your teeth and gums, and how to pick your food astutely for the most ideal oral wellbeing.

Food varieties that invigorate spit creation, advance general oral wellbeing, and give indispensable components like calcium, phosphorus, and nutrients are valuable for teeth. Dairy items, including milk, cheddar, and yoghourt, are incredible suppliers of calcium and phosphorus, two components that are essential for keeping up with the thickness of the jawbone and reinforcing tooth veneer. These food varieties support veneer remineralization, reinforce teeth, and guard against rot.

Since they are rich in water and fibre, crunchy leafy foods like apples, carrots, and celery are really great for your teeth. Biting on these dinners increases spit creation, which supports the remineralization of lacquer, balance of oral acids, and evacuation of food particles and microorganisms. These food sources' crunchy surface likewise works as a characteristic toothbrush, cleaning the teeth's surfaces and disposing of soil and plaque.

Since they incorporate crucial components like calcium, phosphorus, and vitamin D, which are important for keeping sound teeth and bones, nuts and seeds are additionally superb choices for dental wellbeing. Nuts and seeds likewise remember protein and great fats that guide for salivation and guard against gum infection and tooth rot.

At the point when ingested with some restraint, a few beverages may likewise be really great for teeth. Water is the ideal choice for both oral wellbeing and hydration since it keeps the mouth soggy, helps wash away microorganisms and food particles, and keeps up with spit creation. Another astounding decision is green tea, which has cancer prevention agents called catechins that have been displayed to prevent oral microbes from developing and lower the gamble of gum infection and holes.

Nonetheless, certain food sources are inconvenient to teeth and may worsen conditions including gum infection, disintegration, and rot. Sweet food varieties and beverages, like pop, confections, natural product squeezes, and sports drinks, are particularly awful for your teeth since they feed oral microbes, which then, at that point, transforms that sugar into acids that dissolve tooth polish. Over the long run, continuous utilisation of acidic or sweet food sources and drinks could raise your possibility of creating cavities, tooth disintegration, and other dental issues.

Caramel, taffy, and dried natural products are instances of tacky and chewy food varieties that are impeding for teeth since they join to the tooth's surface and stay in the mouth for quite a while, expanding the gamble of holes and rot. Besides, over the long run, acidic food sources and beverages like vinegar, citrus natural products, and tomatoes might dissolve tooth lacquer, making teeth more delicate to rot.

At the point when boring food varieties like bread, saltines, and chips become caught in the little hiding spots of your teeth, they might cause dental issues by filling in as a sanctuary for oral microbes. Subsequent to eating these things, it's vital for brush and floss to dispose of plaque and flotsam and jetsam and safeguard your teeth from future issues.

It is significant to pursue informed food choices to keep up with great oral wellbeing and stay away from dental issues. We might save sound teeth and gums for a long period of grins by decreasing sweet, acidic, tacky, and boring dinners that can add to rot, disintegration, and gum illness and by choosing food varieties that are high in imperative supplements, advance spit creation, and backing general oral wellbeing.

Drinking water for a healthy mouth

Water truly is the "mix of life," as many have said. It is critical for remaining mindful of life and guaranteeing that each veritable framework, including the mouth, has the capacities expected. Staying hydrated all day by drinking sufficient water to maintain major areas of strength and fight against various dental issues is vital.

Washing food particles, creatures, and flotsam and jetsam from the mouth is one of the essential benefits of drinking water for dental flourishing. Food particles and microorganisms could become caught in the space between teeth and along the gum line each time we eat or drink, which can incite plaque variety, discouragement, and gum burden.

Water use helps wash these particles out of the mouth, ensuring oral precision and reducing the gamble of dental issues.

Water is also fundamental for the creation of spit, which is pivotal for dental achievement. Spit prevents dry mouth, a condition that could raise the gamble of dental issues like despairing and gum disease, and lubes up the mouth to make it simpler to tidbit and swallow food. Moreover, spit consolidates minerals and proteins that help dental thriving by remineralizing tooth outsides, killing acids, and crushing perilous microorganisms.

These parts, in this way, thwart weakening and rot.

Fluoride, a routinely occurring mineral present in water sources and dental things, may also cultivate a thriving mouth when crushed in water. Fluoride attempts to upset openings and further cultivate tooth tidiness by ruining the improvement of rot-causing creatures and supporting bits of the tooth that have been compromised. Fluoride is added to different city water sources with the objective that individuals can profit from its benefits for tooth thriving. On the off chance that fluoride is deficient in your water supply, you might need to consider utilising fluoridated toothpaste or seeing fluoride supplements with your dental expert.

Water use also pushes general success and focal flourishing, the two of which impact dental thriving. Different clinical issues, like dry mouth, weariness, cerebral pains, and decreased intellectual ability, might be welcomed by a shortfall of hydration. We can assist with staying away from these issues and save general flourishing and power, which are critical for safeguarding the best dental thriving, by drinking adequate water.

Besides, drinking water is a calorie- and non-sugar substitute for sweet rewards like pop, normal thing presses, and sports drinks, which, when ingested in excess, may incite weight gain and toothache. Picking water as your go-to beverage stays mindful of dental success as well as supports general prosperity and reasonable drinking practices.

Water utilisation is immense for keeping the mouth sound and staying away from dental issues. We can wash away food particles and natural substances, draw in salivation, supply fluoride for tooth cleaning, overhaul general flourishing and flourishing, and look for informed dietary choices that help ideal oral thriving for a critical stretch of sound grins by drinking a lot of water over the course of the day.

Visiting the Dentist

An essential part for kids to protect great dental wellbeing and general prosperity is going to the dental specialist. Customary dental check-ups are fundamental for keeping away from dental issues, recognizing concerns almost immediately, and acquiring master care and treatment to keep your grin sound and brilliant, despite the fact that it's typical for certain people to have an anxious or concerned outlook on visiting the dental specialist.

As well as having your teeth cleaned, you get an intensive evaluation of your oral wellbeing when you see the dental specialist. To search for signs of rot, gum infection, oral malignant growth, and other dental issues, your dental specialist will actually take a look at your teeth, gums, and oral pit. To find any hidden issues that may not be clear to the independent eye, they would also get X-beams.

Prophylaxis, or expert teeth cleaning, may likewise be important for your dental plan. Your teeth will be left perfect and cleaned when a dental hygienist utilises particular instruments to eliminate surface stains, plaque, and tartar. To assist with preventing holes, gum illness, and other dental issues, proficient cleaning is important to eliminate plaque and tartar that can't be disposed of by routine brushing and flossing alone.

Furthermore, seeing a dental specialist empowers you to get redone direction and ideas for protecting the most ideal dental wellbeing. To help you deal with your teeth and gums at home, your dental specialist might give guidance on great brushing and flossing techniques, dietary practices, and oral hygiene items. Furthermore, they might respond to any concerns or requests you could have about your oral wellbeing and give protection estimates like fluoride medicines or dental sealants to fight against rot and depression.

For youngsters, ordinary dental tests are particularly significant since they cultivate serious areas of strength for a dental specialist from the beginning and bestow long-lasting great oral cleanliness rehearses. When their most memorable tooth arises or around their most memorable birthday, kids ought to start going to the dental specialist. Over the course of growing up and youth, they ought to keep on having semiannual tests and cleanings.

With regards to detriment consideration, going to the dental specialist empowers early tooth issue analysis and treatment before they deteriorate. Your dental specialist can treat cavities, gum infections, and other oral medical issues rapidly to prevent further harm and maintain the trustworthiness and wellbeing of your teeth and gums.

Going to the dental expert helps with propelling general flourishing as well as defending dental prosperity. Studies have shown a strong association between principal prosperity and dental prosperity, with sad dental tidiness being related with a higher gamble of respiratory defilement, diabetes, coronary sickness, and different diseases. In addition to the fact that you're putting resources into your grin when you deal with your teeth and gums with customary dental tests, on the other hand, you're putting resources into your general prosperity and life span.

Keeping up with your best oral wellbeing and general prosperity requires customary dental visits. You can ensure a solid, splendid grin into the indefinite future by making an arrangement for ordinary tests and cleanings, seeking master care and treatment, and regarding your dental specialist's exhortation about food and oral cleanliness. Focus on your oral wellbeing and make an arrangement for your next dental specialist visit immediately. Try not to let dread or stress hold you back from getting the vital dental treatment.

Why regular dental check-ups are important

Successive dental assessments are vital for various reasons, a significant number of which work on individuals' overall wellbeing and prosperity. Forestalling dental issues is a significant part. Your dental specialist completely looks at your teeth, gums, and oral pit during a dental examination, looking for signs of rot, gum sickness, oral malignant growth, and other dental issues. Your dental specialist can resolve these issues rapidly to stop more damage and keep up with the honesty and soundness of your teeth and gums by recognizing them from the get-go.

Routine dental assessments empower master teeth cleaning, which is important to dispose of tartar and plaque development that can't be dispensed with simply by brushing and flossing consistently. By dispensing with microorganisms and trash from the surfaces of the teeth and the gum line, proficient cleaning forestalls holes, gum infection, and other dental issues. Proficient cleaning likewise works on the look and newness of your teeth by leaving them polished and clean.

Standard dental exams give customised counsel and ideas for keeping up with great oral wellbeing, notwithstanding precautionary treatment. Your dental specialist might give an exhortation on food, oral hygiene items that are explicitly intended for you, and viable brushing and flossing rehearsals. They can answer any worries you might have about your oral wellbeing and give protection care like fluoride medicines or dental sealants to make preparations for rot and pits.

Besides, kids need to get normal dental assessments since they cultivate a solid association with the dental specialist since the beginning and assist with showing long-lasting great oral cleanliness rehearses. When their most memorable tooth arises or around their most memorable birthday, youngsters ought to start going to the dental specialist. Over the course of growing up and youth, they ought to keep on having half-yearly tests and cleanings.

Successive dental tests additionally support fundamental wellbeing, which upgrades general prosperity. Studies have shown a vigorous connection between foundational wellbeing and dental wellbeing, with unfortunate dental cleanliness being associated with a higher risk of respiratory contamination, diabetes, coronary illness, and other illnesses. Besides the fact that you're putting resources into your grin when you deal with your teeth and gums with ordinary dental tests, on the other hand, you're putting resources into your general prosperity and life span.

Moreover, by keeping away from costly and tedious dental tasks, ordinary dental exams may eventually set aside both cash and time. Your dental specialist can deal with dental worries before they deteriorate and require obtrusive systems or medical procedures by recognizing and treating them at the beginning. This diminishes the monetary strain that accompanies requiring a significant dental fix as well as saving you the misery and burden of going through convoluted dental tasks.

Normal dental assessments are basic for keeping away from dental issues, safeguarding ideal oral wellbeing, growing great oral cleanliness, upgrading general prosperity, and decreasing the time and cost of dental treatment. Focus on your oral wellbeing and make an arrangement for your next dental assessment immediately. Try not to hold on until you're in torment or awkward to see the dental specialist. Your smile will be keen on it!

What to expect during a dental visit

It's normal for children to be intrigued, nervous, or even afraid about what to anticipate when it comes to dental checkups. It's crucial for parents or other adult caregivers to help their children feel at ease and confident during their dentist appointment by preparing them for the procedure.

First and foremost, when children visit the dentist, they should anticipate a kind and inviting atmosphere. Many dentist offices are made with kids in mind. You'll find brightly coloured walls, entertaining games and toys in the waiting room, and kind staff members who specialise in treating young patients. The aforementioned components aim to provide a comforting and upbeat environment for kids, easing any anxieties or worries they may have about dental visits.

Kids may anticipate seeing their dentist and dental hygienist during their appointment, who will put them at ease and welcome them with a grin. Children may communicate their ideas and emotions and take part in their dental care when the dentist asks them questions about their oral health and any worries they may have. Children are encouraged to ask questions and express any concerns they may have regarding the dentist appointment, since communication is essential.

A comprehensive inspection of the child's teeth, gums, and oral cavity is one of the first things they may anticipate from their dental appointment. To make sure that your child's smile is strong and bright, the dentist will use specialized instruments and methods to look for indications of decay, gum disease, oral cancer, and other dental problems. X-rays may be examined as part of this evaluation to search for any underlying issues that may not be apparent to the unaided eye.

Kids may anticipate having a dental hygienist perform prophylaxis, or professional teeth cleaning, after the assessment. The teeth will be left clean and polished when the hygienist uses specific instruments to remove surface stains, plaque, and tartar. To help prevent cavities, gum disease, and other dental issues, professional cleaning is necessary to remove built-up plaque and tartar that cannot be eliminated by routine brushing and flossing alone.

Children may also get preventative treatments like fluoride applications or dental sealants to guard against cavities and decay, in addition to examinations and cleanings. These fast and painless procedures provide your child's teeth with an additional layer of defense and encourage good dental health.

Youngsters ought to expect custom-fitted direction and ideas for saving the most ideal oral wellbeing during their dental arrangement. The dental specialist and dental hygienist will give an exhortation on smart dieting propensities, oral hygiene items that are explicitly intended for your child, and right brushing and flossing rehearses. They could likewise furnish counsel on the most proficient method to manage oral issues such as thumb sucking, pacifier use, and teeth crushing.

In light of everything, youngsters ought to expect a blissful and engaging dental arrangement, complete with kind and circumspect staff individuals who are focused on their oral wellbeing and general prosperity. You might give your child the establishment to a long period of solid grins and charming dental encounters by causing them to feel calm and certain all through their arrangement.

Overcoming fear of the dentist

For youngsters, moving past their feeling of dread toward the dental specialist might be a troublesome yet possible interaction. Kids frequently experience nervousness or anxiety when they are prepared to see the dental specialist as a result of feelings of weakness, apprehension about the obscure, or terrible encounters before. Children may, in any case, figure out how to move past their nervousness and have decent compatibility with the dental specialist in the event that they are given the suitable methods and consolation.

Through training and discussion, kids might overcome their apprehension about the dental specialist, perhaps the most effective technique. Utilising age-suitable language and empowering words, examine with your child what to expect from their dental specialist arrangement. This will assist with mollifying any concerns or nerves they might have. Portray the worth of dental consideration and how the dental specialist attempts to keep up with the strength and soundness of their teeth and gums.

To help your child become accustomed to and standardise the experience of visiting the dental specialist, you could decide to read books or view films about the technique. Currently, there are large numbers of well-disposed young people and materials out there that make sense of dental arrangements in a fascinating and receptive way. Urge your child to share any worries or questions they might have about the experience, and recognize their feelings by giving solace and support.

Steady openness and desensitisation are two more viable techniques for moving past dental tension. First, carry your child to the dental specialist for a meet-and-greet with the dental specialist and staff. This will offer them the chance to investigate the space and become familiar with the sights, sounds, and fragrances of the workplace without feeling hurried or under tension. Plan a progression of brief yet useful dental specialist arrangements. As your youth acquires solace and certainty, dynamically extend and muddle every meeting.

Imagine play and pretending may likewise be helpful techniques for helping youngsters conquer their dental nervousness. Alternate being the dental specialist, dental hygienist, and patient as you pretend a dental arrangement situation utilising dolls, squishy toys, or activity figures. Youngsters might work on survival strategies and critical thinking procedures in a protected and empowering setting with this cheerful methodology, steadily helping their flexibility and confidence.

Kids may likewise be roused and enabled to conquer their apprehension about the dental specialist by getting uplifting feedback and prizes. Recognize your youngster's boldness and collaboration during dental arrangements, and give them a minuscule badge of appreciation or impetuses for completing every meeting effectively. To commend their achievements along the street and monitor their turn of events, contemplate utilising a sticker outline or motivator graph.

Set a genuine example for your family by having an inspirational perspective about dental consideration and planning customary dental exams as a component of their general clinical timetable. Since kids are insightful to parental messages and may get on your concerns, attempt to remain quiet about your terrible words and keep your own dental tension to yourself. Rather, stress the benefits of keeping up with great oral hygiene, the upsides of customary dental tests, and the lovely components of seeing a dental specialist.

Taking everything into account, young people might defeat their anxiety toward the dental specialist with time, empathy, and support. You can assist your kid with conquering their feeling of dread toward the dental specialist and construct a good connection with them for a long period of solid grains by offering schooling and correspondence, progressively uncovering and desensitising, pretending and imagining play, encouraging feedback and rewards, and setting a model.

Caring for Baby Teeth

Dealing with baby teeth lays out the preparation for long-lasting brilliant dental wellbeing and is a vital piece of youth improvement. Albeit temporary, child teeth are fundamental to a kid's overall wellbeing since they advance smart dieting, discourse improvement, and social commitment. Thus, from the time a youngster's most memorable tooth arises, guardians and different parental figures ought to place a high value on oral tidiness and the improvement of good dental propensities.

Keeping up with appropriate oral cleanliness at home is quite possibly the earliest stage in dealing with a baby tooth. Guardians ought to delicately wipe their child's gums with a spotless, wet fabric or dressing after feedings to take out microbes and stay away from the development of plaque, even before the principal tooth shows. Guardians might begin cleaning their youngster's teeth two times every day with a delicate shuddered toothbrush and a spot of fluoride toothpaste as child teeth begin to grow, which is normally close to a half year old enough. To capitalise on fluoride, urge your child to let out additional toothpaste; however, don't wash with water.

For newborn child teeth, flossing is similarly all around as fundamental as brushing them consistently. It disposes of food particles and plaque from the gum line and spaces between the teeth. You might begin utilizing floss picks or youngster amicable flossers to consistently floss your kid's teeth once their teeth contact, which is regularly around the age of a few. While flossing your kid's teeth, use persistence and delicacy. You could likewise have a go at making it a pleasant action by utilising hued flossers or singing a melody together.

Watching out for your kid's eating routine and limiting sweet and acidic food varieties and beverages that could cause tooth rot and holes is one more significant piece of dealing with their child's teeth. Urge your child to limit sweet tidbits and refreshments like pop, desserts, natural product squeezes, and sports drinks, and to eat a balanced eating routine loaded with natural products, vegetables, whole grains, and lean proteins. Rather than taking care of your child's sugar-filled beverages or bites before bed, give them water or milk. This will assist with preventing tooth rot.

Keeping up with great oral wellbeing and dealing with child teeth additionally require ordinary dental assessments. Plan your kid's most memorable dental arrangement for around the hour of their most memorable birthday or when their most memorable tooth is created. Over the course of growing up and puberty, keep on booking half-yearly cleanings and check-ups. The dental specialist for your child can watch out for the improvement of their teeth, spot any potential issues from the beginning, and give protection care and medicines as important to keep a sound and brilliant grin.

Set a positive example for your family by rehearsing legitimate oral cleanliness and focusing on dental considerations in regular exercises. As well as planning routine dental tests for both you and your child, make sure to clean and floss your own teeth consistently. You might set up your child for a long period of solid grins and great oral wellbeing by focusing on the worth of dental wellbeing and ingraining sound propensities at an early age.

Why baby teeth matter

As transitory teeth that ultimately become extremely durable teeth, child teeth—likewise alluded to as essential teeth or deciduous teeth—are imperative to a youngster's development and improvement. They assist with working on a youngster's overall wellbeing and prosperity. Despite the fact that newborn child teeth are only there for a brief time frame, their worth can't be put into words.

The way that child teeth go about acting as guides for the rise of super-durable teeth is one of the primary justifications for why they are significant. For extremely durable teeth to emit into the jaw accurately when situated and adjusted, child teeth help clear space in the jaw. Early tooth misfortune, welcomed on by illness or injury, might make adjoining teeth move into the empty region, which can cause swarming, misalignment, and orthodontic issues from now on. Guardians and different parental figures might diminish the probability that their child will require orthodontic treatment in the future by guaranteeing that their child's teeth stay solid until their extremely durable teeth arise in the legitimate arrangement and position.

Furthermore, baby teeth are essential for smart dieting and processing. Youngsters with sound teeth can effectively nibble, bite, and grind their food into more modest pieces that are simpler to swallow and process. For a sound turn of events and nourishment all through the early stages and immaturity, this cycle is fundamental. Youngsters might feel agony, distress, and inconvenience eating when their child teeth are debilitated by rot or other dental issues. This might bring about dietary shortfalls and unfortunate general wellbeing.

Child teeth are fundamental for discourse improvement as well as filling a pragmatic need in eating and processing. Child teeth's arrangement and position play a part in the improvement of discourse examples and sounds, which let young people articulate words and convey effectively. Youngsters who have absent or lost child teeth might experience difficulty talking successfully, as well as an expanded risk of language deficiencies and discourse disabilities.

Guardians and different parental figures might assist small kids with creating fitting discourse and correspondence capacities by keeping their child teeth in great shape.

Besides, baby teeth support the lips, cheeks, and jaw by helping with the improvement of the face muscles and bone construction. A reasonable and engaging smile is energized by sound teeth and jaws, which support facial evenness and allure. Youngsters might have changes in the design and capability of their teeth, assuming their child teeth drop out too early or are impacted by dental issues. These adjustments might affect the kids' social collaboration and confidence. Guardians and different parental figures might help with their youngster's face improvement and encourage a positive mental self-portrait by keeping their child's teeth in great shape.

The capability of baby teeth to safeguard dental tidiness and wellbeing is another critical element. Like super-durable teeth, child teeth might have depressions and rot, so it means quite a bit to rehearse great dental cleanliness to keep them solid. Normal dental check-ups and cleanings, as well as cleaning and flossing child teeth, may assist with keeping away from dental issues and empowering great oral wellbeing from an early age. Encouraging a long period of sound grins in youngsters might be accomplished by guardians and parental figures by means of the educating of superb oral cleanliness rehearses and the arrangement of suitable dental consideration.

All in all, child teeth are significant because of multiple factors, like assisting with coordinating the rise of long-lasting teeth, advancing sound biting and processing, supporting the advancement of discourse, working on facial appearance, and saving oral wellbeing and neatness. Guardians and different grown-ups who care for youngsters might advance their overall turn of events and give them the most obvious opportunity for a long period of solid grins by figuring out the meaning of child teeth and making a move to keep up with their respectability and wellbeing.

Tips for keeping baby teeth healthy

Keeping up with the soundness of newborn child teeth is essential for advancing suitable oral turns of events and making way for deep-rooted, incredible dental wellbeing. In spite of the fact that child teeth are only present for a brief time frame, they are essential for a kid's solace while eating, talking, and grinning. They likewise go about as impermanent substitutes for the super-durable teeth that will eventually drop out. To keep up with the wellbeing of baby teeth, follow these tips:

1. Start dental cleanliness early on: Your baby might have clean gums even before their most memorable tooth shows up. After feedings, delicately wash their gums with dressing or a perfect, wet material to dispose of microorganisms and prevent plaque from collecting.

2. Tenderly brush: Utilise a delicate, seethed child toothbrush and a spot of fluoride toothpaste to brush your child's most memorable tooth tenderly. Utilise delicate, round strokes to clean their teeth two times every day, in a perfect world, in the first part of the day and not long before bed.

3. Limit sweet beverages: Organic products like juice, pop, and other improved refreshments are instances of sweet beverages that you shouldn't give your baby since they might cause depression and teeth rot. Offer hydration as water, a recipe, or bosom milk, all things considered.

4. Take on great eating practices: Feed your youngster an eating regimen brimming with whole grains, natural products, vegetables, lean meats, and different supplements. Limit how many sweet tidbits and desserts you give them, and avoid taking care of them with chewy or tacky things that could hold up in their teeth and deteriorate tooth decay.

5. Cease making it lights-out time for newborn children with bottles: Cease providing your kid with a container of juice, milk, or recipe to lay down with, as it would cause child bottle teeth to rot. Offer your baby water as opposed to anything else to assist them with snoozing.

6. Sort out for normal dental assessments: Take your child to the dental specialist when their most memorable tooth arises or around the hour of their most memorable birthday. The dental specialist can screen your youngster's tooth improvement and development with routine dental exams, and they can likewise treat and forestall issues as required.

7. Apply fluoride supplements as guided by your dental specialist to fabricate your youngster's tooth polish and prevent cavities. This will depend on your kid's age and dental rot risk. Give close consideration

to your dental specialist's recommendation while utilising fluoride.

8. Advance amazing oral cleanliness rehearsals: Teach your children the benefits of practising legitimate oral hygiene, which includes cleaning and flossing their teeth twice a day and planning incessant visits to the dental specialist. Set a model for others by integrating these schedules into your own regular exercises.

9. Remember getting teeth? It may very well be challenging for guardians and children to go through the getting teeth process. Give your baby a spotless, cool washcloth or getting teeth toys to bite on to help ease their gums. Try not to utilise medications or

get teeth gels without first conversing with your doctor.

10. Stay informed: Find out about suitable dental considerations for babies and small kids by visiting dependable sites, nurturing guides, and paediatric dental specialists. Save up on ideas for taking care of strategies, dental considerations, and oral cleanliness for children and babies.

You can add to the support of your child's teeth and assist them with fostering a long period of incredible dental wellbeing by utilising these ideas and focusing on oral consideration from the beginning. Review that taking great consideration of baby teeth from the outset is critical for solid

nourishment, discourse improvement, and
confidence.

Transitioning to adult teeth

An important developmental milestone for children is when they gradually replace their baby teeth with permanent adult teeth or transition from primary to adult teeth. Children's bodies naturally begin to develop and mature at the age of six, and this process continues until puberty. Although the shift to adult teeth is a typical developmental stage, parents and kids should be aware of the potential changes and difficulties that may arise.

The loss of primary teeth and the emergence of permanent teeth are two of the most obvious signs that a person is changing from baby to adult teeth. Children may start to lose their baby teeth when the permanent teeth beneath them start to erupt as they get closer to turning six. The incisors, or front teeth, normally erupt first, and the molars, or rear teeth, erupt last, usually over the course of many years.

While each child's tooth eruptions may occur in a different order and at different times, most kids will have all of their permanent teeth by the time they are in their early teens. It is crucial that parents and other caregivers keep an eye on their child's dental development throughout this transitional phase and take care of any potential problems, such as delayed eruption, crowded teeth, or impacted wisdom teeth.

Dental discomfort or pain is a frequent issue that kids may have while switching to adult teeth. When permanent teeth emerge, the gums and jaw may experience temporary discomfort or sensitivity, particularly if the teeth are impacted or erupt at an angle. By encouraging their kids to consume soft foods, refraining from chewing on hard items, and maintaining proper dental hygiene to keep the region clean and debris-free, parents may help reduce pain.

The need for regular dental care and maintenance is another facet of the shift to adult teeth. Adult teeth are bigger, stronger, and more durable than primary teeth; hence, they need different maintenance than primary teeth, which are smaller and more fragile than permanent teeth. Using age-appropriate methods and dental supplies, parents should instruct their kids in good brushing and flossing practices to maintain good oral hygiene and stave off gum disease and cavities.

During the shift to adult teeth, regular dental examinations are especially crucial because they enable dentists to track tooth growth, identify any problems early on, and provide preventative care and treatments as required. Starting at age one, or as soon as their first tooth emerges, children should continue to get regular checkups and cleanings every six months at the dentist.

Kids' nibbling and arrangement might change as they become used to wearing grown-up teeth. In some cases, swarming, misalignment, or dispersing issues brought about by the development of long-lasting teeth might be rectified with orthodontic treatment. With regards to their youngster's nibble or arrangement, guardians ought to watch out for their kid's dental development and look for exhortation from an orthodontist.

As a general rule, the method involved with developing into grown-up teeth is an ordinary and regular part of the adolescent turn of events, meaning the improvement of the oral cavity. Guardians might guarantee their youngsters consistent progress and long stretches of good oral wellbeing and grins by giving them the right dental consideration, observing their dental turn of events, and looking for master exhortation when vital.

Protecting Your Smile

For guardians and different grown-ups who care for kids, keeping up with their grins is indispensable in light of the fact that it improves their overall wellbeing, confidence, and general prosperity. A youngster's engaging quality is improved by having a sound smile, which likewise assists with social communication, discourse advancement, and a proper eating regimen. Consequently, it's important to act right on time to shield youngsters' teeth and energise great oral wellbeing.

Imparting great oral cleanliness rehearses in youngsters is one of the most fundamental ways to defend their grins. A long period of legitimate dental consideration is laid by showing kids how to brush and floss appropriately from the beginning. Kids ought to be urged to clean their teeth two times every day for two minutes each time, utilising a delicately shuddered toothbrush and fluoride toothpaste. Furthermore, showing kids how to floss consistently helps safeguard teeth from holes and gum sickness by eliminating food particles and plaque in the middle between teeth.

Guardians might shield their kids' teeth as well as regularly brushing and flossing by empowering a reasonable eating regimen and confining sweet tidbits and beverages. Sugar-filled food varieties and refreshments might compound cavities and tooth rot, so it's critical to train children to pick healthy food varieties and beverages like whole grains, natural products, and vegetables. To protect oral wellbeing, guardians ought to likewise ask their youngsters to drink a lot of water over the course of the day. This is on the grounds that water advances salivation, which is essential for cleaning out food particles and microorganisms from the mouth.

One more fundamental part of protecting youngsters' grins is normal dental assessments. Dental specialists might screen dental development, recognize any issues from the get-go, and give protection care and therapies as required when semiannual arrangements are booked. Proficient cleanings and assessments aid in the expulsion of plaque and tartar aggregation, the location of pits and gum sickness, and the reply to any concerns or requests guardians might have about the oral soundness of their child.

Guardians might shield their youngsters' teeth as well as get ordinary dental care by going to proactive safeguard measures like fluoride medicines and dental sealants. Dental sealants give a boundary against rot on the biting surfaces of the back teeth, while fluoride medicines help to fabricate tooth polish and forestall depressions. Dental specialists endorse these medicines since they are protected, powerful, and suitable for youngsters who have a high risk of pits.

Likewise, guardians ought to protect their kids' grins by monitoring oral propensities and ways of behaving that may be adverse to dental wellbeing. While wearing mouthguards during brandishing exercises stays away from oral wounds and harm, deterring thumb sucking, pacifier utilization, and nail gnawing can assist with forestalling orthodontic hardships and malocclusions. Parental oversight and backing might assist with safeguarding their kids' grins and encourage long-term dental wellbeing and prosperity by tending to these practices at an early age.

All in all, keeping up with kids' dental wellbeing is a perplexing cycle that requires a blend of good oral hygiene rehearsals, a reasonable eating routine, successive dental assessments, precautionary care, and faithful leadership. Parental intercession and proactive measures to protect their kids' grins might assist with ensuring that their youngsters have lovely, solid grins for a long time to come.

Mouthguards for sports and activities

Mouthguards are an essential, however proficient, way to safeguard kids' grins and stay away from oral wounds, making them a fundamental piece of defensive stuff for young people associated with sports and demanding exercises. Whether children are taking part in recreation exercises like bicycling or skating or taking part in physical games like hockey and football, utilising a mouthguard may assist with reducing the risk of dental injury and safeguarding against taken-out or broken teeth, along with other oral wounds.

The limit of mouthguards for youngsters to ingest and scatter influence force during sports-related crashes or incidents is one of its primary benefits. To reduce the risk of mischief to the teeth, jaws, and delicate tissues of the mouth, mouthguards act as a pad between the upper and lower teeth. Mouthguards help stay away from dental emergencies and decrease the requirement for costly and intrusive dental techniques by acting as a defensive hindrance.

Mouthguards may help forestall tooth wounds that can adversely affect children's oral wellbeing and general prosperity. Awful dental wounds might bring about agony, uneasiness, and practical hindrance, notwithstanding surface-level issues and mental misery. These wounds incorporate cracks, separations (took out teeth), and luxations (ousted teeth). Kids may extraordinarily reduce their possibility of experiencing these sorts of wounds and keep a working, sound smile by utilising a mouthguard.

The straightforwardness and versatility of mouthguards for kids are another benefit. To oblige various games and exercises, mouthguards arrive in different structures and plans, for example, stock mouthguards, bubble-and-nibble mouthguards, and custom-fitted mouthguards. To guarantee a cozy and agreeable fit for unhindered versatility and correspondence during play, guardians might pick the decision that best suits their kid's prerequisites, inclinations, and action level.

Mouthguards are low-support and need little upkeep; this assists with broadening their valuable life. At the point when it is not being used, kids ought to keep their mouthguard in a perfect, ventilated compartment, let it air dry completely, and flush it with water after each use. After some time, keeping up with the mouthguard's best insurance and adequacy requires regularly looking at it for wear or harm and supplanting it as needed.

Moreover, youngsters who use mouthguards during sports and proactive tasks might enjoy mental benefits like expanded certainty and smoothness. Youngsters who know about their security against tooth wounds might focus on participating in their number one exercise without agonizing over being harmed. This cultivates an uplifting perspective toward playing sports and keeping up with general wellbeing.

Mouthguards are fundamental prosperity gear for young people partaking in sports and proactive errands, as they provide a direct yet capable strategy for saving their teeth and diverting dental injury. Young people could cut down their risk of dental injuries, keep their smile reasonable and strong, and take part in their main activity with sureness and genuine tranquillity by wearing a mouthguard. To ensure that their children have well-established grins, watchmen and different parental figures should emphasise that their young people use mouthguards every single time a game and amusement works out.

Avoiding harmful habits like thumb sucking and nail biting

It is fundamental to forestall terrible ways of behaving, like nail gnawing and thumb sucking, to keep kids' dental wellbeing at its ideal. Despite the fact that these ways of behaving can initially seem harmless, assuming they are permitted to proceed unrestrained, they might negatively affect dental turn of events and general wellbeing.

Youthful babies frequently foster ways of behaving like thumb sucking and nail gnawing, which are self-calming or strategies for dealing with especially difficult times of pressure or stress. Indeed, even though these ways of behaving could appear to be agreeable for some time, on the off chance that they are not broken from the get-go, they can hurt the teeth, gums, and oral depression over the long run.

The impacts of nail gnawing and thumb sucking on dental arrangement and chomp advancement are among the central concerns. Long-haul nail gnawing or thumb sucking might come down on the jaw and teeth, causing malocclusions, misalignments, and changes in the size and game plan of the teeth. This might prompt nibbles that should be adjusted with orthodontic treatment, like overbites, underbites, crossbites, and open chomps.

Besides, biting one's nails and sucking one's thumb might modify the look and type of the oral cavity, bringing about alterations to the sense of taste, top of the mouth, and tooth arrangement. These modifications might influence a kid's capacity to talk, bite food, and have a satisfying face, which might prompt social troubles and low confidence.

Biting your nails and sucking your thumb could raise your risk of pits, gum illness, and oral contamination. Young people who chomp their nails or sucking their thumbs might bring perilous microbes and microorganisms into their mouths, which can cause gum bothering, teeth rot, and plaque collection. Besides, the power and strain applied to the teeth and oral tissues might bring about scratches, ulcers, and disintegration of the lacquer, making dental hardships almost certain.

Guardians and different parental figures might utilise various strategies to help with solid propensities and support positive options to keep away from and deal with negative propensities like thumb sucking and nail gnawing.

Finding and treating the hidden reasons for nail gnawing and thumb sucking, like weariness, pressure, stress, or frailty, is one technique. Guardians might help young people develop more solid survival strategies for their feelings and diminish their reliance on pessimistic ways of behaving by resolving these basic issues and offering backing and consolation.

Guardians may likewise assist their youngsters with halting biting their nails or sucking their thumbs by utilising encouraging feedback and prizes. Kids might be urged to make positive changes and take up sound propensities by getting commendation and consolation for fantastic achievements, as well as little gifts or motivations for achievements.

Guardians might help their youngsters control their thumb-sucking and nail-gnawing inclinations by utilising conduct intercessions and methodologies. Youngsters might be helped with diverting their motivations and creating substitute survival methods by means of the utilisation of strategies including substitution ways of behaving, interruption procedures, and propensity inversion preparation.

With regards to treating constant nail gnawing or thumb sucking propensities, seeing a paediatric dental specialist or conduct specialist might be useful. These specialists might screen the kid's turn of events, give help in the interim, and make ideas and strategies explicitly take care of meeting their necessities.

It's basic to forestall awful ways of behaving like nail gnawing and thumb sucking in the event that you believe your kid's dental wellbeing should stay at its ideal. Guardians and different parental figures might help youngsters in ending vices, protecting their grins, and advancing long-term dental wellbeing and prosperity by tending to these ways of behaving at an early age and utilising social mediations, uplifting feedback, and master support when important.

What to do in case of dental emergencies

In order to protect the child's safety and wellbeing in the case of a dental emergency, parents and other caregivers must maintain composure, evaluate the situation, and take the necessary action. Dental crises may happen quickly and without warning and can be brought on by trauma, accidents, or the abrupt onset of excruciating tooth pain. Parents who are prepared for such scenarios can handle the emergency and tend to their child's needs quickly.

A knocked-out (avulsed) tooth is a frequent dental emergency in children. It's critical to take immediate action to save a child's tooth if it has been knocked out by stress or injury. This is what you should do:

1. Remain calm and comfort the youngster.

2. Find the tooth and treat it with caution, holding it by the crown (top), not the root.

3. Use milk or a saline solution to gently rinse the teeth if they are filthy. Use no soap, water, or other cleaning solution to scrub or clean the teeth.

4. Attempt to put the tooth back into the socket, making sure it faces in the proper direction. To keep the tooth in place, have the youngster bite down gently on gauze or a clean towel.

5. If reinsertion is not an option, keep the tooth moist by placing it in a

container of milk or saliva. The sensitive cells on the root surface may be harmed if the tooth is kept in water.

6. Get dental treatment right now. As soon as you can, try to get in touch with the child's dentist or go to an emergency dental clinic within half an hour after the damage.

An additional frequent dental emergency in children is a shattered or broken tooth. Take the following actions if a child's tooth is broken, chipped, or cracked:

1. Use warm water to rinse the child's mouth in order to clear any debris and disinfect the region.
2. To lessen discomfort and swelling, apply an ice pack or cold compress to

the area of the mouth next to the damaged tooth.

3. If at all possible, save any broken tooth pieces; your dentist may be able to repair them.

4. Make an emergency dental appointment by calling the child's dentist. Explain the circumstances and provide any pertinent information about the injury.

5. As instructed by the kid's doctor, give the child over-the-counter pain relievers such as acetaminophen or ibuprofen if they are in excruciating discomfort.

Dental emergencies in children might include things stuck between teeth, acute toothaches, abscesses, or soft tissue damage.

To treat the problem and relieve the child's pain and suffering in any of these scenarios, it is imperative to seek dental care as soon as possible.

Guardians ought to find proactive ways to forestall dental emergencies by ensuring their children wear mouthguards while playing sports, ceasing from gnawing on ice or hard articles, ingraining great oral hygiene practices, and making continuous arrangements for cleanings and tests.

Guardians and different parental figures should know what to do if a kid has a dental crisis. Guardians may effectively deal with dental emergencies and ensure their children seek speedy attention and treatment to protect their oral wellbeing and prosperity by keeping calm, assessing what is happening, and making the fundamental move.

Fun Interactive Activities to Reinforce Oral Hygiene Habits

One of the best ways to build a lifetime commitment to dental care and maintain oral hygiene practices in youngsters is to include them in enjoyable and engaging activities. Parents and other caregivers may empower kids to take charge of their oral health and help them form good associations with dental care by making oral hygiene fun and engaging. Here are some imaginative and enjoyable exercises to help youngsters practise good dental hygiene:

1. **Storytelling:** Write a lighthearted and inventive tale with characters that place a

high value on dental cleanliness. Introduce ideas like brushing, flossing, and going to the dentist in a lighthearted and approachable manner by using stories. Invite kids to join in by having them play out situations, create sound effects, or write original tales with a dental health theme.

2. Brushing and Flossing Games: Add entertaining tasks, timings, or prizes to brushing and flossing to make it into a game. Make it a game called "toothbrushing bingo" where kids have to complete each phase of their oral hygiene regimen to win stickers or prizes, or challenge them to brush for two minutes while dancing to their favourite music. Similarly, urge kids to "rescue" their teeth from "cavity monsters" by using coloured dental floss and having them floss in between each tooth.

3. Interactive Apps and movies: A plethora of instructive applications and movies are accessible to educate kids about dental care in an engaging and interactive manner. Examine interactive applications with games, animated characters, and music on flossing, brushing, and going to the dentist. You may view these movies and applications as a family or let the kids explore them on their own.

4. Oral Health Crafts: Use your imagination to create crafts that promote good oral hygiene practices. Allow kids to personalise their toothbrushes or toothbrush holders by using glitter, paint, or stickers. Establish a jar labelled "tooth fairy" where kids may gather missing teeth and give them to the tooth fairy in return for a little gift. Additionally, you may create a "toothbrushing chart" on which kids can use stickers or bright markers to record their regular brushing and flossing schedules.

5. Role-Playing Games: Get kids to act out various dental situations, such going to the dentist or taking care of their teeth at home. To make the experience more realistic and engaging, give them fake playsets, dress-up costumes, and toy dental instruments. Children may get used to dental practices and treatments via role-playing in a secure and comforting setting.

6. Oral Health Workshops: To educate kids about good oral hygiene, arrange interactive workshops or lectures with a paediatric dentist or dental hygienist. Under the supervision of a dental expert, let kids ask questions, take part in demonstrations, and practice brushing and flossing procedures. Provide youngsters with practical exercises like brushing models or revealing tablets to demonstrate successful plaque removal.

7. Family Challenges and contests: Set up friendly contests or challenges within the family to make dental hygiene a game. Try putting family members to the test to see who can floss and clean their teeth the best or longest. Establish a "smile jar" where kids may win prizes or benefits for regularly maintaining proper dental hygiene. As a family, celebrate successes and milestones to support one another's good conduct.

Parents and other caregivers may help kids associate dental hygiene with pleasure and rewards by including these engaging activities into their schedules. Children who are raised with a favourable attitude toward dental care from an early age are more likely to form lifetime habits that support the best possible oral health and wellbeing.

Oral health puzzles, quizzes and Games

Oral wellbeing puzzles, tests, and games for youngsters are engaging as well as instructive, giving a tomfoolery and intelligent way for kids to find out about legitimate oral cleanliness propensities, dental considerations, and the significance of keeping up with sound grins. These exercises connect with kids' interest, imagination, and critical thinking abilities while building up key ideas connected with oral wellbeing and dental cleanliness.

One famous sort of oral wellbeing game for youngsters is puzzles, which challenge kids to take care of issues, match shapes, or complete pictures connected with oral wellbeing themes. For instance, kids might be entrusted with gathering a riddle portraying a toothbrush, toothpaste, and dental floss to build up the significance of brushing and flossing consistently. Riddles can likewise highlight pictures of sound and unfortunate food sources to show youngsters the effect of diet on oral wellbeing and urge them to pursue better decisions.

Tests are one more captivating method for testing kids' information on oral wellbeing ideas and supporting key learning targets. Tests might incorporate various decision questions, valid or bogus articulations, or fill-in-the-clear activities connected with brushing methods, pit anticipation, and dental life structures, and that's just the beginning. Kids can go up against one another or challenge themselves to acquire focus and compensation for the right responses, making finding out about oral wellbeing fun and fulfilling.

Games offer intelligent and active opportunities for kids to investigate oral wellbeing ideas in a fun, loving, and drawing way. For instance, youngsters might play a memory matching game where they coordinate pictures of sound and undesirable food sources with their comparing impacts on teeth. Different games might include pretending situations, for example, claiming to be a dental specialist or dental hygienist and performing dental check-ups on dolls or toys. By taking part in these games, kids can acquire a more profound comprehension of oral wellbeing themes while improving their social abilities and imagination.

Intuitive applications and online stages offer an extensive variety of oral wellbeing games and exercises planned explicitly for youngsters. These computerised assets frequently include beautiful illustrations, energised characters, and intuitive components to catch kids' attention and keep them locked in. Youngsters can investigate virtual universes, complete difficulties, and procure prizes for finishing oral wellbeing-related errands like cleaning their teeth, flossing, and eating good food sources. Guardians and parental figures can download these applications or access them online to enhance their kids's oral wellbeing instruction and support great dental propensities at home.

Integrating oral wellbeing puzzles, tests, and games into kids' everyday schedules can make finding out about dental consideration more agreeable and paramount. These exercises give diversion and feeling as well as enable kids to play a functioning job in keeping up with their oral wellbeing and creating deep-rooted propensities that will uphold sound grins into the indefinite future. By making oral wellbeing instruction fun and intuitive, guardians, teachers, and dental experts can rouse kids to focus on their dental wellbeing and make informed decisions about their oral consideration propensities.

Conclusion

"Oral Health Book For Kids" is more than just a book—it's an entryway to a long period of blissful lips and solid smiles. Youngsters go on an astonishing excursion to find out about the worth of ordinary dental check-ups, the need for good oral cleanliness rehearsals, and the role that sustenance plays in dental wellbeing by means of spellbinding stories, intelligent riddles, and engaging games. This book gives kids the data and cutoff points they need to deal with their oral flourishing and use great impulse about their dental thoughts, from pressing brushing procedures to dumbfounding flossing works out.

Past its convenience, nonetheless, this book provides messes with a healthy identity worth and confidence by exhibiting to them that they are fit for monitoring their prosperity and grinning. "Oral Health Book For Kids" constructs the establishment for a long period of sound grins and cheerful mouths by empowering great mentalities toward dental consideration and solid ways of behaving since the beginning.

Kids will find out about oral wellbeing standards and dental life structures as they turn the pages of this book; however, they will likewise track down the joy of dealing with others and themselves. They assume the job of promoters for their own dental wellbeing, empowering others to esteem dental consideration and perceive the engaging quality of a certain, splendid grin.

So could we go out on this experience together and research, make, and advance as we uncover the favoured bits of knowledge of oral prosperity? We might find the keys to a long period of sound grins and set out a way to an existence where each youngster can grin with certainty and enjoyment by utilising "Oral Health Book For Kids" as our aide.